The Juicing Bible

Second Edition

Pat Crocker

Robert
ROSE

The Juicing Bible, Second Edition
Text copyright © 2000, 2008 Pat Crocker
Photographs and illustrations copyright © 2000, 2008 Robert Rose Inc.
Cover and text design copyright © 2008 Robert Rose Inc.

This is a revised and expanded edition of *The Juicing Bible*, published by

For complete cataloguing information, see page 366.

Disclaimer
The Juicing Bible is intended to provide information about the preparation
whole foods and medicinal herbs. It is not intended as a substitute for prof
publisher and author do not represent or warrant that the use of recipes or
in this book will necessarily aid in the prevention or treatment of any disea
any liability, loss or risk, personal or otherwise, incurred as a consequence,
and application of any of the contents of this book. Readers must assume so
lifestyle and/or treatment program that they choose to follow. If you have qu
of diet and health, speak to a healthcare professional.

The recipes in this book have been carefully tested by our kitchen and ou
our knowledge, they are safe and nutritious for ordinary use and users. For th
allergies, or who have special food requirements or health issues, please read
each recipe carefully and determine whether or not they may create a proble
at the risk of the consumer.

We cannot be responsible for any hazards, loss or damage that may occur a

For those with special needs, allergies, requirements or health problems, in
please contact your medical adviser prior to the use of any recipe.

Design and Production: Joseph Gisini/PageWave Graphics Inc.
Editors: Carol Sherman and Sue Sumeraj
Proofreader: Karen Campbell-Sheviak
Indexer: Gillian Watts
Photography: Colin Ericson
Photograph of Tomato Juice Cocktail: Mark T. Shapiro
Photograph on chapter openers: istockphoto.com/arsat
Food Styling: Kathryn Robertson and Kate Bush
Prop Styling: Charlene Ericson
Illustrations: Kveta/Three In A Box

Cover image: Strawberry Sparkle, see page 204.

We acknowledge the financial support of the Government of Canada through the
Development Program (BPIDP) for our publishing activities.

Published by Robert Rose Inc.
120 Eglinton Avenue East, Suite 800, Toronto, Ontario, Canada M4P 1E2
Tel: (416) 322-6552 Fax: (416) 322-6936
www.robertrose.ca

Printed and bound in Canada

11 12 13 TCP 18 17 16 15 14 13 12